Newly revised

REBECKA VIGUS

So You
THINK
You Want
to Be a
MOMMY?

a guide for teens and adults

ZANDER

Livonia, Michigan

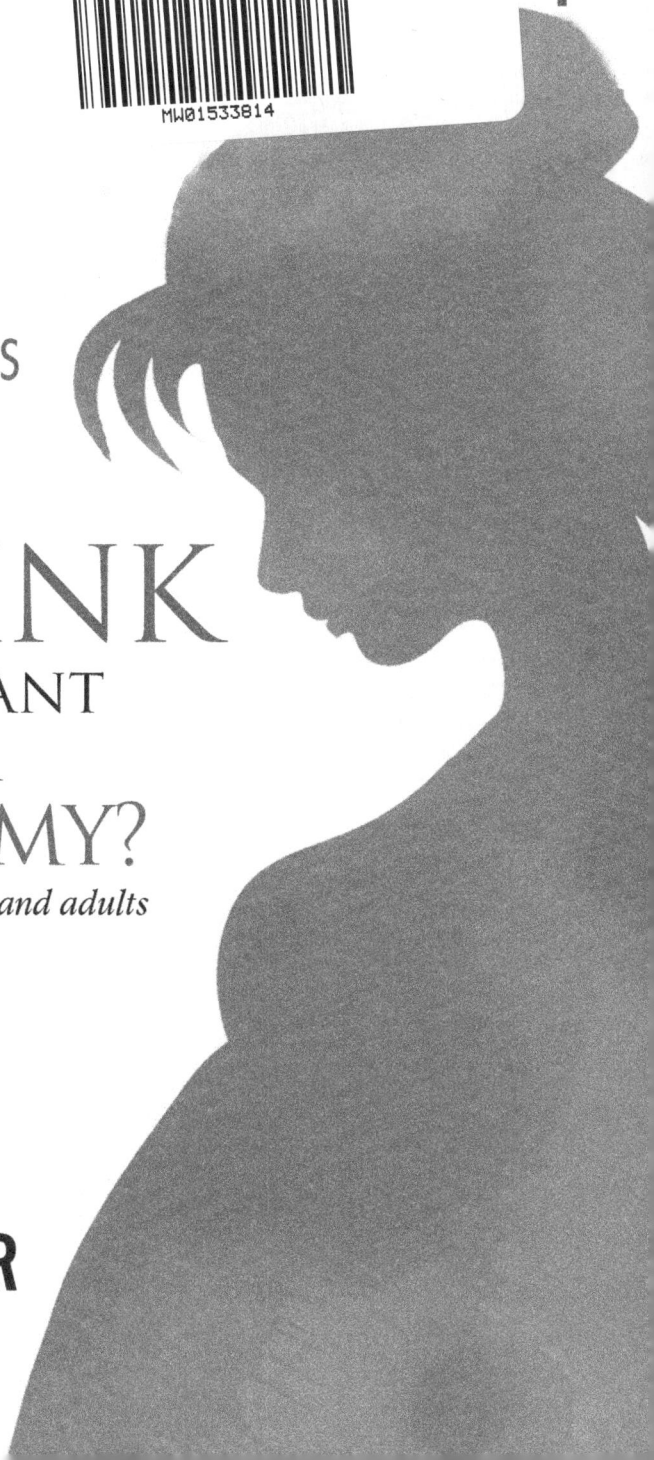

Published by Zander
an imprint of BHC Press

Library of Congress Control Number:
2017945126

ISBN-13: 978-1-946848-47-5
ISBN-10: 1-946848-47-6

Visit the author at:
www.bhcpress.com

Also available in ebook

ALSO BY REBECKA VIGUS

FOREWORD

I did my student-teaching at an inner city high school in Flint, Michigan. After I did some substituting in the same building, I was flabbergasted when during the last week of school the young single mothers dressed up their babies and brought them to school. Having at baby at the time, 1986, was thought to be a status symbol.

I was a single mom at the time. My daughter was in fourth grade and I didn't understand the concept of babies being status symbols. It was as if these young girls thought they had to prove they were women.

Well, it's now 2017 and it frightens me to hear the young girls talking about having babies. They have no clue what they are in for. I do and I wasn't a teen when I had my daughter.

This book does not discuss sex or the precautions one should take to have safe sex. This is a book about some of the things which can happen to you when you get pregnant and are single. It's all about the things you won't find in those beautiful baby books. Those might be able to tell you what to expect physically and I'll leave it to them. This book will tell you some of the emotional upheavals you might face, some of the stress you might come under, and will ask you some very serious questions.

If you are even thinking about having a baby and you are still in high school or just out of high school, please read this book. Listen to the stories of the moms I talked with. Is this where you really want to end up? Is this the future you have planned? Wouldn't it be better to wait until you are married and have a stable home to provide?

Rebecka Vigus

This book is dedicated
to the ladies who took time to
share their stories for this book.
Without them, there would be no book.

Thank you, Ladies.

So You THINK You Want to Be a MOMMY?

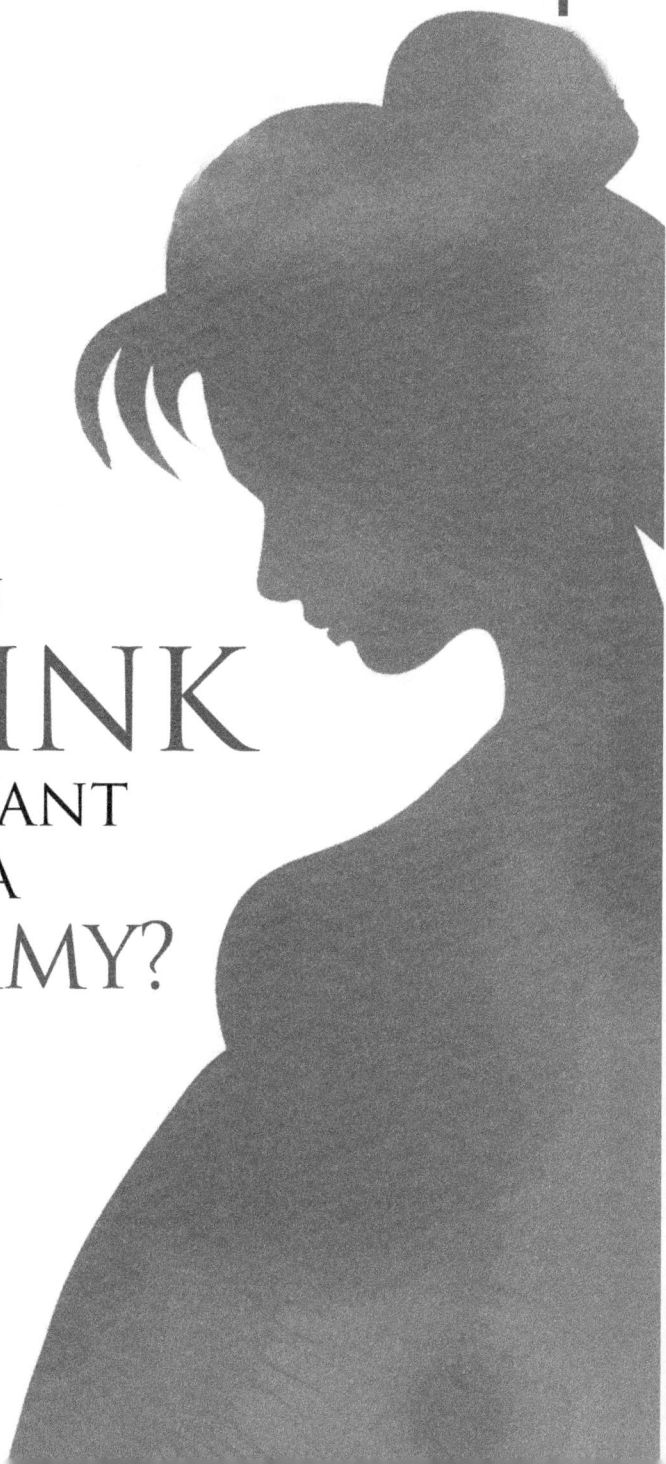

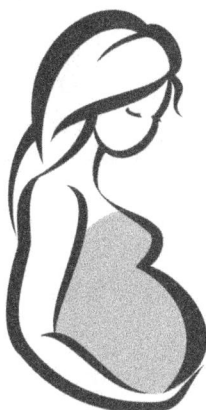

INTRODUCTION TO MOTHERHOOD

So, you think you want to be a mom. The first thing you should consider is; does your boyfriend want to be a dad? Are you old enough to get married in your state? Have you discussed children? Do you feel like this is the only thing which will keep you together? Is he pressuring you for sex? Have you talked about STDs? Have you talked about what will happen if you do get pregnant? Are either of you working? Are you finished with school?

Still think you want to be a mom? Well, let me tell you all the things you won't read in a baby book. Starting with you will now be taking on a full-time 24/7 job. Do you realize this job is for life? It doesn't stop just because you get bored. It continues until you die. How old are you? If you are sixteen, you are looking at approximately sixty years on the job and there is NO retirement plan, there is NO income to rely on. Your rewards will come only with the success of your child. If your child fails, of course, you will be blamed. Children don't come with manuals. Are you ready for someone who is totally dependent on you?

What about your social life? Well, if the guy sticks around and you get married, you have someone to share the job with. But, don't hold your breath for it to happen. Most guys your age aren't ready to take care of themselves let alone a wife and child. They still want to party with their friends. Where will it leave you? At home watching the baby, of course. There is no guarantee he will get up in the night if the baby is ill or that he will even change a diaper. Does this wonderful guy even have a job? There is also nothing to say you won't divorce down the road. There are no guarantees in this life. You can forget dating. He doesn't want to be seen with you either. Although just yesterday he was defending your honor. If some other guy does ask you out, he is probably looking for a one night stand. Most guys don't want to be saddled with a child. Still sound glamorous? What about your girlfriends? They'll treat you like you have THE plague. You won't get invited to parties, shopping, or just to hang out. They'll be too busy shopping or hanging out with their boyfriends to have time for you. Feeling lonely yet?

Loneliness is something you will need to get used to. You cannot have much of a conversation with an infant. You will get bored reading the same story over and over again, or playing the same game. You'll get tired of trying to sound happy about your best friend's latest boyfriend, her new job, or the outfit she just bought at the GAP. Not many people will be dropping by to see how you're doing after the first month or so. There are days you will be bored to tears. No one to talk to, all your friends busy, just you, the baby, and the diapers.

Have you thought about where you will live? Your parents might be willing to take in you and the baby, but they don't have to take in your boyfriend (especially if you're not married). Are his parents going to want you and the baby? Maybe before, but things have changed. There is a new opinion of you. All of a sudden, you're a tramp, it doesn't matter if you were a *nice* girl yesterday and his parents loved you. The baby is not his. He's not taking the responsibility for this mess. His mother claims you trapped him, even if you had a good relationship with her before the pregnancy.

Remember you always have to face your parents. What plans did they have for you? College? Career? No doubt they will be disappointed. How much are they willing to support you? Will they toss you out on your own? Are you a minor? Will they want you to have an abortion or give the baby up for adoption? Will they want to raise the baby as their own? Oh, no!! What will you do? How could you do this to them? How will they ever face the neighbors? The people at church? What were you thinking? If you don't think there will be ranting and raving you are sadly mistaken. This guy they liked last week will be the bum who has taken advantage of their little girl. They will want you to break up with him. They will also want him to act responsibly and pay medical bills and child support. And there you will be caught in the middle. Are we having fun yet?

Your figure you've been so proud of is now gone. If you're lucky you might be able to see your feet when you deliver, but I wouldn't count on it. How was your health before pregnancy? Will you have gestational diabetes? Will your baby be premature? Do you smoke? Have you been drinking? How are your eating habits? Will you gain too much weight? Getting your figure back and keeping it will become another life-long job. There will be diet and exercise. Oh, more never ending jobs.

Are you still in high school? This could pose a problem. Will the school let you attend regular classes or do you have to attend an alternative high school, or will you be considered a homebound student? How are you going to finish all your classes so you can graduate? Did you have a career in mind? How will you accomplish it? Who will watch the baby while you are in school? How are you going to study and raise a child? More problems you didn't consider. They just keep coming, don't they?

Sleep. Have you thought about it? Get all the sleep you can now, because in a few months you won't be getting much. You'll have to get up for a night feeding and usually a diaper change. You will be up bright and early for feeding and a diaper change. You will be up every time you hear your child whimper. You will walk the floors at night if your baby has gas, colic, or a temperature. Your baby might have its days and nights mixed up. You will find yourself falling asleep when your baby naps during the day, just to stay alert at night. There won't be anyone to do these things for you. There you are, alone again.

How will you support your child? Diapers aren't cheap. Don't count on the daddy. Even if you get a child support order, you may not see child support. Did you know a baby goes through a diaper an hour to begin with, except while sleeping at night and then it should only be two diapers...the one it goes to bed in and the one you change it into at 2 a.m. feedings. Did you know it costs approximately $18,000 a year to raise a child? Let's see $18,000 times 18 years, hmmm... approximately $324,000 and we haven't even discussed college or major medical issues. Hope your savings account is full. What no savings??? Where are you going to get that kind of money?? Grandma and Grandpa don't have to foot this bill.

Daycare. Have you thought about it? Have you considered the cost? You might be surprised to find out grandmas don't want to be tied down with a baby. They have raised their children. They may help once in a while, but don't take them for granted. How are you going to find good daycare? How will you know your child is safe? You cannot always count on a daycare facility to have good staff they only pay minimum wage, but you will pay an arm and a leg. Depending on where you live, a day care center can run from $200 to $500 a week. Some of them don't take babies. Some don't take children who are not potty trained. If you go to in home daycare, you can expect to pay from $100 to $300 a week. That, too will depend on where you live. Will you have to supply diapers? Usually and only disposable. Will you have to supply food? If your child is still taking a bottle, you will probably have to provide them as well as beginning food. Some centers charge more if they are providing food. Some in home daycares ask you to provide cereal or bread on a weekly or bi-weekly basis. Have you allowed for this? Will you be eligible for public assistance for daycare? How much will you have to pay out of pocket? Remember that may limit where you can take your baby, too. For in home daycare are you able to do a background check on the person providing the service? How do you know this will be a safe environment for your child? Remember your child will be spending a lot of time in a daycare setting. It won't be home, but your child should be safe and you should not have to spend your day worrying.

Also when you are considering daycare, you want to look at the opportunities they will provide your child. Will your infant be held? Will anyone read to your child? Are they just baby-sitting or will your child have age appropriate educational experiences? Are they making sure your child doesn't get hurt? Will there be pre-school opportunities when your child gets older? What kinds of things will they be teaching? Are there academics? What do they charge if you have to work late?

You might want to check the first aid background of the people taking care of your child. Do they have any first aid training? How do they handle accidents? Are they going to call you at work for every little thing? Are they going to tell you how your child got bruises or scrapes? These are things you might want to know. What are the procedures for someone else picking up your child? Do they check I.D.? Are there only certain people who can pick up your child? What happens when your baby is sick? Daycare doesn't have to take sick children. What is your alternative plan?

Do you have medical insurance? Does your doctor take Medicaid? Do you know there are doctors who don't? Do you have a regular doctor? Is this the same doctor who will check your baby? Do you know about the shots your child needs and when they need them? What if your child is born with a birth defect or serious health problem and requires surgery or special care? Those bills can be staggering to anyone. How will you cope? Do you plan to breast feed or bottle feed? Have you looked at the cost of formula? WIC only covers certain kinds. Are you applying for welfare? Is this how you want your child to grow up? Will you apply for WIC? Do you even know what it is? Are you seeing anyone on a regular basis who can help you through all this? Your DSS worker really doesn't care. He/she has 100 other people to account for. Have you gone to a crisis center? Do you have a birth coach? What if there are complications during pregnancy which will affect your health? Or the baby's health? It may sound like twenty questions, but these are some things you need to consider.

Are you considering adoption? Have you contacted an attorney or agency? Do you know exactly what your rights are? Will you be selecting the family or is someone else doing it for you? If you are selecting the family, are they paying any of your medical bills? Have you received permission from the father to allow the adoption to go through? Is he fully aware of his rights? Does he have his own attorney? What a mess this can become. Do his parents want to raise the child? Is he going to fight you for custody? Getting confused? Does your head hurt just thinking about it?

Are you considering abortion? Do you know what an abortion is? Do you know there can be complications? Are you going to a clinic? Have you talked to a counselor? Are you going to be able to live with this choice? Have you talked to a minister, priest, or rabbi? Have you checked into the cost? Do you know if this is the right decision for you? How does the father feel about this?

If you have considered all of this and still want to have a baby, talk to someone whose been a single mother. How did they do it? How did they cope? Did they finish school? Do they have a job? Do they feel trapped? Do they consider themselves successful? What is the age of their child? Do they have more children? What have they given up? What would they do differently? Would they have made different choices? What regrets do they have if any?

Let me tell you about being a single mom. It has been the most rewarding thing I've ever done. It has also been the loneliest and hardest choice I've had to live with. The story goes like this:

I was dropped from student-teaching five weeks before my college graduation. My world was collapsing. I scrambled to find a job. I ended up as the secretary/receptionist for a ballroom dance studio. This was a whole new world for me. I had never considered being a secretary, not that I thought less of people who became secretaries. I had always wanted to teach. I was shell shocked and trying to learn something new. I didn't have a clue as to what a cutthroat business ballroom dance was. It was there I met Mr. Wonderful. He was a dance instructor. He was seven years older than I and charming. He was also divorced with two little girls. He swept me off my feet. He had dinner with me and took me dancing after work. I couldn't believe he was attracted to me. I'd been working there about four months when he asked me to marry him…and tumble into bed. We put matching wedding bands in lay-a-way and I was hooked.

When I discovered I was pregnant, my world went spinning out of control. I was thrilled. Mr. Right informed me he was still married… oops did he forget to mention that? Also, he had a live-in girlfriend. She was a new twist. And I shouldn't expect any money from him. Gee, wasn't that a surprise? What in the world was I going to do?? Now I was getting scared and I hadn't even told my parents yet.

I was living in an apartment. I had a job. I had meager savings and insurance which did not cover pregnancy. What was I going to do?

I finished college and ended up on the unemployment line. I did get $50 a week in unemployment...now that was going to go a long way—NOT. I was eligible for food stamps, of course, I had to pay for them. Mr. Right had disappeared. This was not what I planned for my child or myself for that matter.

I still had to tell my parents. As I expected it was awful. They were NOT pleased. I continued to look for work, but no one wants to hire you when you are pregnant.

The pregnancy was easy. My daughter was born the Saturday after Thanksgiving in the early hours of a rainy morning. I had complications requiring a blood transfusion. I spent four days in the hospital and returned to live at my parents. They had come to accept they were going to be grandparents and did give me support.

I had two friends who stuck by me during all of this. One was male and became my daughter's unofficial uncle and her father figure for the first six and a half years of her life. The other was my best friend from college. She was always there, even though she was starting her new life. My friends from high school??? They're out there somewhere. One had the nerve to get mad at me because I didn't tell her beforehand I was having a baby. We don't even talk now. Over the years, I've reconnected with some friends from college, but my friends from high school are pretty much gone. My childhood friends are still around.

When my daughter came into the world I had no job and $15 in the bank. I made her formula from scratch...a mixture of Karo syrup, water, and condensed milk. I also used cloth diapers. (Disposables were out of my price range). I started looking for work when she was a week old...I actually got a job when she was two months old. I worked crazy shifts. It was hard to hire a sitter, because I never knew from week to week what my schedule would be. I changed jobs six months later. My new job was an office job… I was an employment agent finding other people work. I was paid a draw against commission. (For those who don't know what that means. I was paid a weekly salary and when my commissions came in they would take them for what they had already paid me). I was there about four months. My last pay from them was $30.00. Then I was hired at a small manufacturing company as the receptionist. It was a great job. I had a regular schedule and a steady income. Surprise…after a year, the company downsized and I was laid-off. It took me two months of standing in unemployment lines to find another job. This one in a hospital pharmacy. A job which lasted over seven years and helped me buy my first home. A job I came to hate.

I was lucky. I lived with my parents the first four years of my daughter's life. I started paying them rent after I had been working six months. (Even parents have the right to charge rent).

I was also lucky to have a brother and two sisters who helped make sure my daughter didn't lack for anything. My sisters pitched in to baby-sit and my brother taught her to be a tomboy. She was always surrounded by love. I was granted a child support order in October, 1977, almost a year after the birth of my daughter. It was to be $25 a week. Which didn't even cover the $40 a week in daycare. Of course, it didn't come either. I didn't get child support until my daughter was 28. You do the math. Gee, where was this money when I actually needed it? With interest and penalty fees it was almost double what it would have been had it been paid on time. It should have been paid off in about fifteen years. She would have been 43 by then. Unfortunately, her father died in September, 2015 still owing child support.

She met her father for the first time when she went to college in the town where he lived. She was almost eighteen. Imagine her shock to learn she had seven younger half siblings. She knew about the four older half-sisters, because I had known about them. Her dad fathered fourteen children we know about. Four of her siblings were deceased, both sets of twins. Imagine her father went on to have another family and *never* tried to find out anything about her. What an eye opener for an only child who had always wanted brothers and sisters. Does she respect her father? No, but he is her father.

I am a successful person. I hold a Bachelor of Science Degree, a Master of Arts in Teaching, and all but the thesis for an Education Specialist Degree. One I am most likely not to finish. I taught school for 28.5 years, 22 in special education. I've raised a beautiful daughter who is still the center of my world. Has it been lonely? Yes. Many times, I've sat at home while friends have gone places. They often ask me to accompany them, however I hate being the fifth wheel. Do I wish I'd found someone who was Mr. Right? Yes. Have I become self-reliant? Yes. Do I know I have family I can count on? Yes. Are there things I would have done differently? Only in my relationship with her father…I'd have taken more time and really gotten to know him. Of course, if I had, I wouldn't have my daughter. Do I regret the choice I made? NEVER. Do I recommend the same choice for others? No. I personally think in this day and age no girl or woman should find herself in this situation. There are too many ways to prevent it.

Update on where I am. I have found Mr. Right, he was standing in front of me all my life. Don't take your best friend for granted. I am an author of three ebooks, two novellas and one almost in print, five novels, this book which comes under self-help, one poetry book and I'm working on a novel and a writers' workbook for a class I plan to teach. I also own my own publishing company and sponsor three authors with one more on the way.

I don't want anyone to get the idea this book is about me. It's not. I went and talked with others who were and are single moms or found themselves pregnant and unprepared. The following are their stories, I hope you will gain some valuable insight from these extraordinary women. They made mistakes, they are not perfect, they were not prepared, they handled their unplanned pregnancy in their own way, and not all of them lived happily ever after.

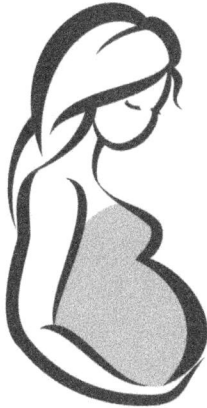

TIFFANY

She was twenty when she met Mr. Right at work. She'd finished high school and had some college. She'd been dating Mr. Right two and a half months when she got pregnant. The only children they had talked about were the two he already had. He reacted by telling her, "Fall down the stairs and get rid of the problem." If she was unwilling to do it, he would be more than happy to help. Their relationship was over within a month of learning she was pregnant.

Her parents and family were disappointed, but supportive. Tiffany was frightened every step of the way during her pregnancy. First, she worried about being HIV positive. (Mr. Right liked to sleep around). Once she crossed that hurdle, she faced others.

She lost many of her friends. Some just didn't understand at all. She did manage to hold on to a few.

Tiffany considered abortion, however once she heard the baby's heartbeat she could never have gone through with it. She also knew she could never carry a baby nine months and then give it away. It was scary and stressful. She was thankful to have such a solid support system.

She chose not to seek child support. She did not want to put her child in a position of seeing a father who didn't want her or might abuse her.

Postpartum depression hit Tiffany hard after the birth of her daughter. In her words, "The depression after her birth was unbelievable. The first few days after she was born, I think I was just numb and really tired. By about the end of the first week or early into the second week, I was convinced I was not capable of being a mom. It seemed like nothing I did made her happy. She cried constantly and never wanted me to put her down. On top of that, she didn't take to breast feeding and I felt like a major failure. Luckily the severe depression only lasted a couple of weeks, but it was so bad at one point, I told my mom I was going to sign over custody because I couldn't do it."

She was only a single mom for a year and a half. It was the hardest job she's ever had, but also the most rewarding. She was scared most of the time and never seemed to have enough money. Thankfully, her mom helped her out a lot and she had assistance through WIC.

Tiffany encountered frustration when taking her daughter to the pediatrician, especially when her mom came along. If mom was there the doctors talked to her instead of Tiffany, treating her as if she weren't even there. It made her feel like she was incapable of taking care of her own child.

When asked if she could do it over again, would she get pregnant? She responded it was a loaded question. Would she have been more careful? Yes. Would she change the fact she had her daughter? Not ever.

At this point in her life, Tiffany is in what she describes as her "beautiful place." She's been happily married for almost five years and has two beautiful children. Her husband adopted her daughter, warming everyone's heart. She's successful in most ways. She has finished college. As far as marriage and parenting go, she's a smashing success. She works a full-time job and two or three part-time jobs, her husband works full-time. Yet both of them find time for family.

This is not something she wants for her daughter or her son. She feels anyone who wants a baby young is a fool. You have to give up your own childhood and you miss out on so many things in life which are important at a young age.

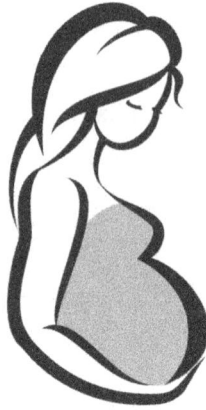

SARAH

S arah was nineteen and had been in a relationship for three months when she discovered she was pregnant. In any conversation, they had about children, Sarah was sure she didn't want any. The initial shock was hard. They didn't know how to talk or react to the situation. As a result of the pregnancy she grew closer to Mr. Right. They eventually married.

She found herself unsure all the way through her pregnancy. Her friends didn't want to talk to her. She was no longer invited to parties.

Her mom took the pregnancy okay. Her family has been real supportive when she needed help. She worried about having enough money, but knew her family would be there if she needed things. She watched her mom raise her as a single mother (her parents divorced when she was an infant) and knew everything would work out.

Sarah says she wouldn't change anything and has no regrets. She's very successful, has finished college. She feels she has a wonderful family with two children.

Pediatricians treated her differently. Once she even changed doctors because of the way she was treated. She says when trying to rent an apartment she ran into the same thing.

Sarah's advice to teens and young women is: "Be a kid! Don't have a baby until you are ready. Go to college and have fun. With kids, you miss out on a lot of things.

Update on Sarah. She married her Mr. Right. They now have a daughter and a son. She has her own business in real estate. Life is good.

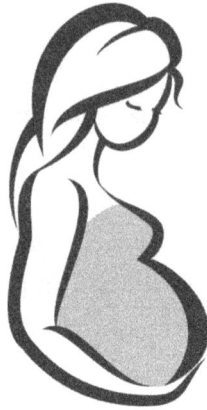

JENNIFER

Jennifer was sixteen when she learned she was pregnant. She'd been in a relationship for just over two years. They discussed kids, but for some time in the future. Her relationship with Mr. Right went down the tubes.

Her mom cried when she got the news, but her dad said, "I told you so." She had enough friends and family for support to not be frightened during her pregnancy.

Most of her friends just accepted her situation. One friend said she, "knew" Jennifer had gotten pregnant on purpose. Then didn't speak to her for quite a while.

Jennifer's friends and family were great at watching her baby, so she could finish school. She graduated with her class.

She says she has no regrets, but if she could do it over, she wouldn't at the age she was. Her daughter sees her father regularly, but Jennifer didn't get child support until her daughter was seven.

Jennifer sees herself successful. She is a stay at home mom with an eleven year old daughter, a two year old son and a baby on the way. She has her own business designing houses from her home. She found her Mr. Right and they have been married four years.

Jennifer has no regrets, but getting pregnant was not a decision she made consciously. She loves her daughter dearly and all she brought into Jennifer's life. She would never change a thing, but she can honestly say, she would not have tried to get pregnant just because she thought it was "cool." This is not something she would want for her daughter.

She doesn't remember how she felt as she was a pregnant teen and teen mom. When she found out she was pregnant, she knew her life would be drastically different, but she accepted the consequences of her carelessness. She didn't dwell on the things she was not able to do; starting college right away, go out with friends, etc. Abortion and adoption were not options for her.

Her advice to teens thinking about having kids, would be to ask them to think about their lives right now and all the freedoms they have. Then imagine all or most of those freedoms gone. Would they like giving up all the "cool" things they are free to experience now? Then ask them to look ahead to the future. Where do they see themselves in five, ten, or fifteen years?

An update on Jennifer. Her daughter was seventeen when she announced she was pregnant. Jennifer was not pleased. She is now the mother of four, two girls and two boys. She still works from home.

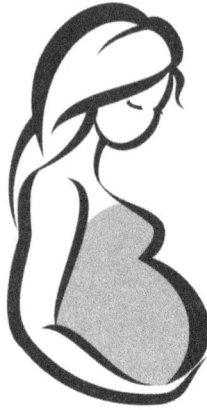

TRISTA

Trista was twenty when she became pregnant. She had not been in a long-term relationship and they had not discussed children. She was a high school grad, but had to drop out of college, which was as devastating for her as it would have been if she'd dropped out of high school.

Raised by her grandpa she was most worried about telling him. He was a pastor, so had a great deal of grace and forgiveness and it wasn't as bad as she thought it would be. She was exceedingly scared to tell him. She was lucky and he loved her through it all.

As to her relationship with Mr. Right, she ended up leaving him the night she told him she was pregnant. His first reaction was, "Are you getting an abortion?" She told him, 'NO WAY!" He was upset about it. They got into an argument and Trista left. It was a few months later she talked to him, but they never got back together. They are however, civil to each other.

Trista was scared all through her pregnancy. She was lucky and had good friends who helped her make the decision to drop out of college and come home. She is aware some family and friends look at her differently.

She was stressed throughout her pregnancy, but she had friends and family to support her. Even though she was not with the baby's father, he did help support her. She didn't have to pay rent for a while, she qualified for WIC for the baby formula, and she was working full-time. Still she found the money did not stretch to pay for everything she needed. It was stressful even in the good times.

She didn't worry about taking care of the baby and going to school, since she dropped out of college. When she was pregnant she was living off student loans she had. She didn't work for a couple of weeks, then got a job so she could start saving. Before her little daughter was born she moved into the basement of the baby's father's house. She kept her job the entire time she was pregnant. After having the baby, she took a few weeks off then went back to work. Her daughter's grandmother watched the baby while she worked.

If she could do it over again, Trista would take precautions so she didn't get pregnant. When asked if she has regrets, Trista says sometimes she regrets leaving her daughter's father the night she told him and other times she regrets talking to him again. She definitely does not regret having and keeping her daughter. She thinks her daughter's life would be different if she had stayed and worked things out. She sometimes regrets talking to him after going their separate ways, as it's hard for her daughter to go back an forth to her dad and step-mom's every week.

Her daughter sees her dad weekly. She does not get support for her daughter. For the first six months, she was living in his house and then she moved to her own apartment. Whenever she needed money he gave it to her. They split everything in half as far as clothes, extra-curricular activities, etc. Since Trista got married in February, 2008, she has received no child support.

Trista is now happily married with three children, her daughter and two sons. They have gone from renting from her mother-in-law to owning their own home. Her husband has a good job and Trista does photography in addition to her full-time job.

Her advice for teens who think it would be "cool" to have a baby is; "Cool...Are You Crazy??? There is nothing "cool" about raising a child when you are a child yourself." She was older when she had her baby, but it was still hard.

She is glad most of the time, her daughter has a relationship with her father, but she feels it would have been easier for her and her daughter, if he were not a part of their lives. Her daughter going back and forth between them is the worst part of her situation. She thinks her daughter has everything she want for her...four loving parents, lots of grandparents, aunts, uncles, and other family members who love her. Trista always thinks it could have been better, but this is the way it is and God has blessed her.

Her final thoughts to share are at the time of pregnancy she never thought she could make it through. She had a lot of help from both sides of the baby's family and friends. She also had God, whom at the time she had strayed from. She has started her relationship with God and it is how she got to where she is. Many young moms are not as fortunate as she was and she feels she has God to thank for it. She guesses her advice for young women wanting to get pregnant is, "Find God and GREAT support system, because it may be possible to do it on your own, but she had a lot of support and still had a hard time she couldn't have made it through on her own.

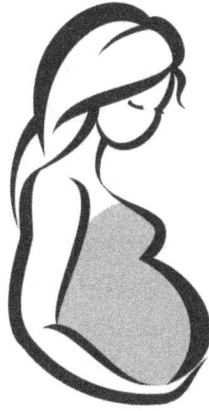

BARB

B arb was fifteen when she found herself pregnant. She had been in a relationship for two years. They had talked about children, but she was too young to understand what they were talking about. Her pregnancy was a combination of carelessness and planning, although at her age it was a careless decision.

Her mom had died, but her dad was angry when he heard about it.

Barb was frightened throughout her pregnancy. She ended up quitting school. Her friends treated her differently. She had no one to turn to for advice. She got married, but her husband became lazy and abusive.

Barb loves her children, but would be more careful if she had it to do over again. She has lots of regrets.

Barb's children do not see their father and she does not receive support. She was always worried and ended up giving her kids up for adoption. She had a daughter with medical problems and she didn't have health insurance. She was only a child herself with three kids in diapers. She was depressed and felt lost. When she decided to give her kids up for adoption, she was mad at herself, but knew it was what was best for them. They needed a stable home.

Her first three children were with her first husband. She was able to pick the family who would raise her children. Two other children were with her current husband and again she got to pick the family who has them. She is able to exchange letters with the adoptive family and they send her photos of the kids. Last summer she had an opportunity to see her youngest daughter.

She finally feels successful. She got her GED and is enrolled in college. She also works full-time.

Her advice to young girls is to consider what it is you are willing to give up, including your children.

Barb lost the job she had and has dropped out of sight.

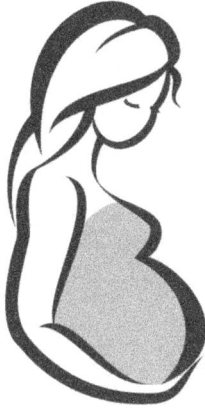

AMY

A my was seventeen when she got pregnant. She had only been with her Mr. Right for a month. They had never discussed children. This was carelessness on their parts.

She was not living at home at the time so, it's really hard to know how her parents felt about her pregnancy.

She had her daughter the summer between her junior and senior year of high school. Mr. Right was a lot of help while Amy was finishing school. They took turns getting up in the night and he took care of the baby so she could go to school. She was able to graduate with her class.

Mr. Right stayed with her for two years for the baby. Amy doesn't think they were ever in love.

She was scared the entire time she was pregnant. In fact, so scared she didn't think she'd make it through the pregnancy.

Amy's friends treated he differently. It's hard to find things to do with your friends when you have a kid to bring along.

If Amy could do it over, she would be more careful and not get pregnant so young. As to regrets, it's a hard question for her to answer. She wouldn't change anything now, because she loves her daughter.

Mr. Right has been a big part of her daughter's life and Amy feels they're lucky. She continues to get support for her daughter.

Now Amy is happily married to someone else. In addition to her daughter, she has a son, two step children and a child on the way. It's been ten years since she graduated and it's much easier being pregnant this time.

When asked if she feels successful, Amy says, "Not yet, but I'm working on it." She feels like she is on her way.

Being a single mom made her grow up real fast. When she left her daughter's dad, she was the only one to support them. She had to work two jobs to support them. She did it! She never let her daughter go without. She worked hard to make sure she could do it.

Being a single mom is a lot of sleepless nights and hard work. Not everyone has the help Amy had. Her advice is, "Wait until you're older and ready for responsibility."

This is not what she wants for her daughter and hopes her daughter will learn from her mistakes.

Amy does not believe in abortion; however, she did consider adoption. Then she felt her baby move and knew it was out of the question.

Update on Amy: Her daughter is a college graduate and has already entered the work force. She has her own apartment and says she doesn't want to be like her mom. She paid attention to the lessons she learned.

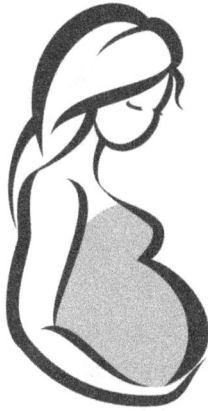

MEGHAN

Meghan was twenty-one when she learned she was pregnant. She and her Mr. Right had been together about a year. They had not talked about children. This was a surprise for them as Meghan was on the pill. She figures she is part of the 2% it doesn't work for.

Her parents took it a lot better than she thought they would. They were disappointed in her, but within two weeks were excited and making plans.

She is still with her Mr. Right. Although they are together they have their ups and downs. It has been an adjustment period, because they don't get to spend time alone like they did before.

Meghan was scared during her pregnancy about how they were going to financially afford a child. She was scared Mr. Right would leave, but he has stayed around and been a big helper. She still worries about money, but they seem to always come out okay, even if it means she and Mr. Right do without. She has learned to use the resources available through the Family Independent Agency and WIC.

She learned very quickly who her real friends were. She lost friends because they didn't understand she couldn't go out just any time. Most of the friends she has now, also have children. Her guy friends reacted better and have stayed around.

Managing to study has been hard. Although Meghan finished high school, she was trying to continue her education. She also had to learn to manage her time. She does a lot of studying at night when her daughter is sleeping.

If she could do it over again, she would. Adoption and abortion were never considerations for her. She has no regrets. She gets a lot of support from her daughter's father and the baby's super grandparents and godparents.

Right now, she working and going to school. She feels successful. She has continued to go to college and will graduate in 2005. Her daughter is growing, learning, and happy.

Although this is not what she wants for her child, she will support her not matter what happens.

Meghan's advice to young women considering pregnancy is they should wait. "Children are expensive and time consuming. High school should be fun and somewhat carefree. It should be all about dances and friends. Having a baby changes it all and it's better to wait."

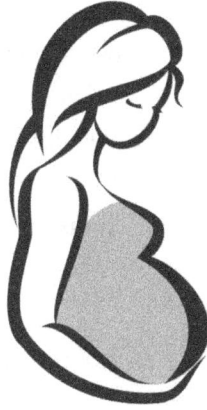

POTENTIAL HEALTH RISKS

Okay, are you convinced yet? Do you still think having a baby is the answer? There's more. Have you thought about all the things which can go wrong during pregnancy? Let me tell you about a few. The list is not complete, nor is it intended to replace medical care. I am not a physician, but I do know these are some things which can go wrong during pregnancy.

Ectopic Pregnancy

This is when your egg is fertilized in the fallopian tube. It is very painful and generally leads to a miscarriage. If you have an ectopic pregnancy, you need to seek immediate medical attention. Medication can be given if the fallopian tube is not ruptured. If it has ruptured, you need immediate surgery. It will leave scar tissue on the fallopian tubes and might make it hard to get pregnant in the future.

Miscarriage

Miscarriage, is the natural loss of a child. It usually happens in the first trimester, but can happen later. What will your feelings be if this happens? Will others tell you it's for the best? Will you continue your relationship with Mr. Right? Will you try to get pregnant again right away? You will suffer grief. This is the loss of a person.

Gestational Diabetes

This is when your body cannot produce enough insulin during your pregnancy causing you to become diabetic. Usually it is discovered between twenty-four and twenty-eight weeks. It puts you at high risk for high blood pressure during your pregnancy. If you have it in one pregnancy, you are at risk for later pregnancies, and could develop Type II Diabetes in the future. You will need to eat a balanced diet throughout your pregnancy. You will need regular exercise and to monitor your blood sugars. Your doctor should help guide you through this. You might have to give yourself insulin, hope you aren't afraid of needles. You will also have to monitor the baby's movement and notify the doctor if there are changes. Do you know how this might affect your baby? How will it affect you after the baby?

If you are diabetic when you get pregnant, you have a whole different set of issues. You need to work closely with your doctor to prevent issues at the time of delivery.

Premature Birth

Premature birth happens later in your pregnancy. It could be caused by trauma, such as a car accident or it could happen naturally. Will the baby survive? Will it have life threatening health issues? Will the health problems continue throughout the child's life? How will you pay for this? How will you cope with this?

Placenta Previa

This is when the placenta is delivered before the baby. It usually happens in the twentieth week of pregnancy, but can happen later. It can first be noticed as vaginal bleeding. Depending on how much bleeding you are doing it could be monitored as an out-patient or you could be hospitalized and receive blood transfusions. This could cause birth problems for the baby, as it could get tangled in the umbilical cord. The baby could die in this situation. To prevent this a C-section is usually performed.

RH Sensitivity

This happens if you have a negative RH factor in your blood and your baby has a PH factor in theirs. The mother's immune system produces antibodies to destroy the baby's red blood cells. Each pregnancy makes the problem worse. Have you even heard of the RH factor?

Pre-Eclampsia

This is when you have high blood pressure during pregnancy. There are underlying reasons for pre-eclampsia. First, a family history of pre-eclampsia. Second, it occurs most often in women having their first baby. Pregnancy may trigger something in the woman's immune system causing high blood pressure. Third, might be the mother's body reacting to the placenta. Finally, underlying problems with kidneys or diseases affecting the blood can cause it. Close monitoring by your doctor will be necessary. Diet, mild aerobics, and blood pressure medications can also be used in the treatment of pre-eclampsia.

Hemorrhage

Hemorrhage or uterine bleeding happens in some women after delivery. It can be very frightening. It is the third most common cause of death in new mothers. It happened to me. They had to get an anes-thesiologist up to delivery to put me out, so the doctor could pack my uterus and stop the bleeding. I remember thinking as I went under I was going to wake up having had a hysterectomy. It didn't happen. However, in the waiting room, my parents had been told I had the baby and would be out to see them shortly. An hour later, my parents were still waiting and they were sure one or both of us had died. No one had taken the time to tell them I had complications. I was rather groggy when I saw them in the recovery room and told them they had a granddaughter. It was a frightening time for everyone.

If none of this has an effect on you, then consider what could happen to your baby. If you smoke, you are likely to have a low birth rate baby. Great, you're thinking, you won't look fat. Wrong! You may not look fat, but your baby could be born prematurely and with under developed lungs.

Other Medical Conditions

Do any partying while you were pregnant? Ever heard of **Fetal Alcohol Syndrome?** It's the effect alcohol has on your unborn child. The extent of the damage will depend on how much and how often you drink and the child's genetic susceptibility and how far you are in your pregnancy. Five or more drinks at any one time can cause growth retardation, facial abnormalities, mental retardation, behavior, and learning problems. If you drink less than five drinks during your pregnancy, you might find your child has these symptoms only milder. Alcohol may cause premature delivery, miscarriage, or still birth.

Are you a teen? You are at risk for having a **Low Birth Rate** baby. This means your baby may weigh less than 5.5 pounds. It also means some of your baby's organs may not be fully developed. This can lead to lung problems like respiratory distress syndrome, bleeding in the brain, loss of vision, and serious intestinal problems. Babies with low birth weight are more likely to die in their first year of life than normal weight babies.

Also, if you are a teen, your body is not fully developed. Pregnancy can put unnecessary strain on your pelvis causing permanent damage. You are at risk for high blood pressure and stroke.

There's also **Spina Bifida**, which is when the babies spinal cord does not develop correctly. It might grow outside the baby's body requiring immediate surgery after birth. Surgery to close an opening may be required. Sometimes the baby's urine will have to run through a bag which needs to be changed regularly. This can be mild or severe. Are you ready to handle a special child? Do you have family and financial support to care for a child with this kind of medical need? Some children with spina bifida also have water on the brain requiring surgery to insert a shunt to drain excess water from the brain.

What about **Cerebral Palsy?** This is a brain trauma to your baby before or during birth. It is more common in premature or low birth weight babies. Again, are you emotionally ready to handle a baby who is not quite "normal?" There are degrees of cerebral palsy. Some cases are so mild you wouldn't know unless you were told. Other cases are severe and anything in between. How are you going to handle this?

Don't forget about **STDs.** You may be carrying one right now and not even know. There are at least thirty STDs now. We do NOT have cures for those which are viruses. Some of them can permanently damage you. Some can actually kill or be passed to your child during birth. Just a few more complications to be worried about. If you are sexually active, pregnant or not you need a regular pelvic exam. Even if it means telling your mom. Do it for your own health. Do it for the health of any children you might have in the future.

There's only one more thing you haven't considered, I'm sure. What if you have multiple births, say twins or triplets? That's double everything. Do you think you will be able to feed and change two babies in the middle of the night? What kind of trauma are you facing now? Even if you have some hope of supporting one child, can you even consider two or more?

You've read our stories, you've read some of the risks and you still think you want to have a baby? Ask yourself these questions first and answer them honestly.

1. What's happening in your life?
2. Do you need to find someone to help you cope with it?
3. What are you running away from?
4. What support system do you have to help you with your problems?
5. Is a baby really going to make things better?
6. Or is having a baby going to create more problems?
7. Are you having a baby to spite your parents?
8. Are you having a baby to hang onto your boyfriend?
9. Are you having a baby because your best friend has one?
10. Are you having a baby so someone will love you?
11. Better yet, what can you offer a baby?
12. Are you able to provide a home for it?
13. Are you able to prepare a baby for college?
14. Are you able to handle the 24/7 responsibilities which accompany a baby?
15. Can you be assured your baby will not grow up in poverty?

16. What does your future look like without a baby?

17. What does your future look like with a baby?

18. Have you picked out a career?

19. Can you get to your career choice with a baby?

20. Are you ready to talk to someone about which choice you should make?

Here we are finishing up twenty questions. Unlike the game Twenty Questions, these are meant to be serious and you need to look closely at your answers.

Most communities have crisis pregnancy centers. Find yours before you get pregnant. Planned Parenthood is one of those. They have counselors who will talk with you throughout your pregnancy, however, they would like to talk to you before your get pregnant.

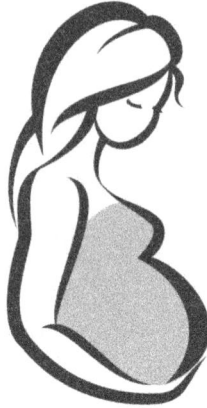

SUPPLEMENTAL ARTICLES TO READ

For those of you thinking about having a baby, you might first take a good look at your relationships. There are several relationships you need to look at. Let's start with your parents.

How do you get along with your parents? Are on good terms with them? How could your relationship with them be better? Do you live with both parents? If your parents are divorced, do you play one against the other? Be honest, many children do this with their parents. It's much harder if your parents are still married. How long have your parents been married? What is good about their relationship? Have you talked to them about relationships? Ask your mom how she met your dad. Ask your dad the same question. Ask them how they feel about each other today. Is it different from when they were first dating? When they were first married? These are some things you might want to know.

Now, let's look at your relationship with your boyfriend? How long have you been dating? Have you had sex yet? Has it been protected sex? How many other guys have you dated? Take a long hard look at this young man of your dreams.

Get a piece of paper; fold it down the middle length ways. On the left-hand side, write all the good things about him. On the right side, write all the things you don't like about him. Does he smoke? Drink? Party every week-end? Drive recklessly? Do drugs? Swear constantly? Does he hit you or belittle you? Has he finished high school? Does he have a job? What are his manner like? Does he attend church or have any religious beliefs? Think long and hard about him.

Next, what is your relationship with his parents? Do you even know them? What are they like? Do they like you? Do you feel comfortable around them? Would you be comfortable spending a lot of time with them? Remember they will be your child's other grandparents. Are they good with kids? Talk to his mom about how she met his dad. Are you even comfortable talking to her? It might be a good idea to make another list of likes and dislikes.

Now you have some lists and have had some time conversation. (Or at least I hope you've had some conversation and made some lists). It's time to talk to Mr. Wonderful. Does he want children? If so, when? Does he even like children? Can he support them? Is he ready to make a life time commitment? Look at your list of things you don't like about him. Many of these things you won't be able to change. Harping and nagging will not make a difference. (Most likely he will want to spend more time hanging out and partying).

Put your lists away. I want you to make a promise to yourself, you will not get pregnant or push the issue of commitment for six months. At that time, take out your lists and look at them again. Are there any changes you want to make? Do it. Have there been changes in your relationship? Have you changed?

If after six months you still think he is Mr. Wonderful and you have no major changes, find someone you trust to talk to. This could be a teacher, counselor, clergy, best friend, parent, parent of a friend, but it needs to be someone you can really trust. Show them your lists. Talk about them and about the lists. See what they have to say. Maybe they have more questions for you. Listen to them.

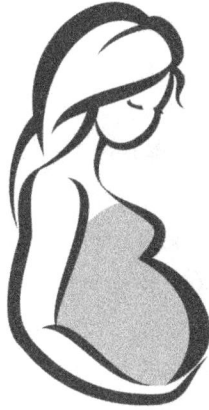

RELATIONSHIPS

B y definition a relationship is: A particular type of connection exist-ing between people related or having dealings with each other.

Whatever you think, it doesn't happen overnight. Relationships are built over time. You have to start with some common beliefs or interests. You have to learn the habits of the other person in the rela-tionship. What do they like? What do they dislike? How do they get along with your friends and family?

I have many relationships. Some are better than others. Some are for business reasons. Some are personal. Each one of them takes time and effort. Left alone, they would dissolve and finally disappear.

My best girlfriend and I have been friends for over forty years. We met in college and have been through a lot together. We have different religious backgrounds and different political beliefs. We don't focus on our differences. We focus on the things we enjoy doing together. It's wonderful to spend a day shopping, having lunch, taking in a movie, or just hanging out. We've even traveled together. She introduced me to Las Vegas and slot machines. I take her with me on road trips via telephone and computer. She is starting to take her own road trips.

We have also struggled with relationships. Hers with her late husband and mine with my parents and my daughter. We have been there for each other. We've lost friends together which is heartbreaking.

If I were to stop calling her, spending time with her, or sending her emails, I am sure we would both find other ways to spend our time. We would both probably wonder what happened, but we'd move on. She plays devil's advocate to me when I have a new idea. She challenges the things I want to do, so I can make sure they are the right things for me. I'm never sure I bring as much to the relationship, but I try.

We met in my first semester of college. I'm not quite sure why the relationship took. We were in the same dorm and often met for breakfast. She was much more studious than I was. She was the steady one in the relationship. I was more the "let's do it now" person. It seemed to balance for us. She graduated two years ahead of me. I felt lost with her not there, but wrote letters (we didn't have computers or cell phones, they hadn't been invented). I have a collection of drawings she used to put on my letters and envelopes. I probably spent more time in the library my last two years, because her study habits wore off.

After forty plus years there are still new things I learn about my friend. She never ceases to amaze me. Once she took a job on a toll bridge where she was required to climb to the top of the bridge to open it. I never wanted a job that bad.

As for courage, she has more than anyone I know. She faced cancer alone. She quit her job to take care of herself. She drove herself to chemotherapy and home again. She never asked anything of anyone. She didn't want a fuss made. When she was diagnosed, she got on the Internet and found out everything she could about the type of cancer she had. She was a fountain of facts and information. When she lost her hair, she found wigs...let me tell you she rocked her wigs. When her hair grew back in curly, she found ways to make it work for her. She is always on alert for a return of the cancer.

She's deeply religious. Her whole life is built around her faith. No matter what is thrown her way, she has her faith to see her through.

I didn't learn this in a month or even a year. It has taken over half a lifetime to learn these things. Long term—lasting—relationships take time to build. They take nurturing and effort in order to stay strong. You need to be ready to work at it.

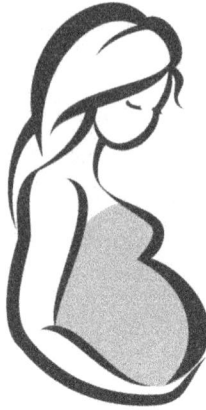

UH, OH. FOUND YOURSELF PREGNANT?

O kay, so you found out you're pregnant. Who do you tell first? The baby's father would be the logical choice. Your parents would be next. The question is, how are you going to tell them? If you just found out, no one knows. You need to spend a little time absorbing the fact and thinking about how, when, and where you are going to make this announcement.

Your Parents

Doing it during an argument is not the time. Doing it at the dinner table is not the right time. Telling them to be spiteful is not the right time. So, when is the right time? You need to make this decision. It needs to be done tactfully and you need to show maturity when you tell them.

Your Boyfriend

Announcing to your boyfriend in front of all his buddies would not be a good time. Telling him the next time you are getting ready to have sex is not the right time. You need to choose your time and place carefully. It will never be a perfect time, but some times and places are better than others. He should probably know before you tell your parents and definitely before you start telling your girlfriends. He might want to go with you when you tell your parents. He might want to tell his parents the same time you are telling yours. Pick a quiet time for this serious talk.

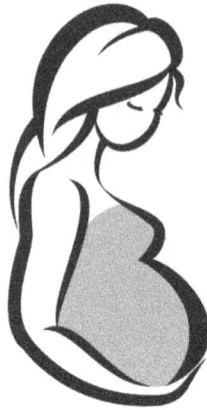

SINGLE AND PREGNANT:
WHAT TO DO NEXT

Okay, so you're single, pregnant, and scared. What happens next? There are several things you need to do and soon. One is to see a doctor. Work out a payment plan if you don't have insurance, but see a doctor. This will help your pregnancy go smoothly and your baby to be healthy. Find someone who can go along with your; your mom, a close friend, someone who can help you when you don't understand what is happening to your body. Someone you trust, who can take notes for you, who will be a sounding board if you have questions.

If you don't take care of your health, your baby has less chance of being healthy. If you smoke, stop. DON'T drink. I don't care what your friends say. It will affect your baby and they won't be around when you have to deal with those problems.

Still talking to the baby's dad? Ask him how much he is going to help you with expenses. Find out if he has insurance which will cover you. Find out what your parents are willing to help with. It won't be everything. They raised you. You might even have siblings they are still raising. Assess your resources, then look for where you can get help.

Crisis pregnancy centers are there to give you assistance, use them. Don't be afraid, they are not going to judge you.

Tell your parents. They may be disappointed, but they are still your parents. Be sure your boyfriend tells his parents. This will be their grandchild, too. They might want to help.

Know your emotions will be on a rollercoaster. One minute you will be laughing and the next you will be crying and not know why. Look at all your options to make the best decision for you and your baby. Don't panic. You will get through this. Take it one day at a time.

Are you old enough to work? Have you finished high school? Can you really keep this baby? Do you understand what it means if your boyfriend walks?

Option 1

Have an abortion and go on with your life as if the pregnancy never happened. This will take some soul-searching. Can you live with killing a child? That's what abortion is.

Option 2

Keep the baby and raise it yourself. You do realize most children with single parents grow up in poverty. Often the cycle of poverty repeats itself. You could find yourself a grandmother in sixteen years.

Option 3

Give your child up for adoption. This is another soul-searching option. Is giving your child up in the best interests of the child? Can you live with someone else raising your child? What kind of adoption do you want? Would it be open where you would have an opportunity to see your child? Would it be closed where you would not know what happened to your child unless he/she decided to look for you at some time in the future?

Option 4

Have the child and let your parents raise it. It is another form of adoption.

Option 5

Give full custody to your boyfriend and his family to raise. You may or may not have visiting rights or pay child support. It is something determined by the courts.

None of the options is an easy choice to make. Make lists of the pros and cons of each. Option 1 has a time limit on it, so you have to decide quickly.

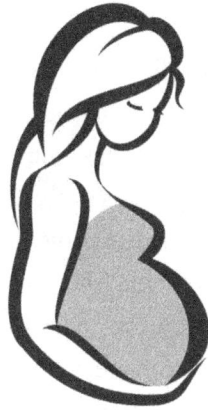

PARENTS…IS YOUR TEEN HAVING SEX?

I s your son or daughter a teen? Has he/she started having sex? Who is providing birth control and what is being provided? I know girls as young as thirteen and fourteen who are having sex. Some with single partners, other with multiple partners. Some are using condoms, some are using birth control pills, some have the depo shot, some have IUDs, and still others are having unprotected sex. Oral sex is still sex.

Samantha and Jeff had been "going together" since the start of their eighth-grade year. By November, they were the talk of the school. Samantha thought she was pregnant. Jeff was trying to figure out how he was going to keep going to school and find a job to help pay for a baby. The sad part of this story, they had not had sex. They had come close, but had not truly had sex.

Pregnancy is not the worst thing which can happen to your child. When you were a teen, there were four STDs and they could be treated with a round of antibiotics. Today there are over thirty STDs and many of them are viruses. There is no cure and antibiotics will not solve the problem. Did you know of the twenty-six new STDs, twenty-two of them could kill or maim your daughter? There are some your daughters could get, with will not be discovered until she is married and wants to have children. Endometriosis is one of those. It destroys the fallopian tubes, preventing eggs from getting to the uterus…no babies. Sometimes it even requires surgery to remove the uterus.

AIDS is not just a homosexual disease and the age group it is rapidly growing among is teens. There is NO cure for AIDS. Sometimes people don't even know they have AIDS for up to ten years.

Know where your children are, who they are with, and what they are doing. Sex is not a game. It is not uncontrollable. But, you cannot look the other way. Your daughter's boyfriend should not spend the night at your house, nor should she spend the night at his. This is just an invitation for trouble. Be the parent. You can be their friend when they are adults. Know what is going on with your child. Talk to your child about sex, STDs, AIDS, and the other consequences of having sex too young. Don't let them be Samantha or Jeff.

The entire episode with Samantha and Jeff (not their real names) blew over, however not before the damage was done. They are no longer even friends. Both are still in school and both have totally different outlooks on relationships. Living in a small town has not helped. They cross paths on a regular basis. He has chosen not to use Facebook except to play games. She uses it as gossip central. They have done some growing up and much faster than they should have. Mostly because no one ever talked to them about sex and the responsibilities that go with it.

Don't let this be the story of your child. Talk to them early. Explain the dangers and the responsibility. Don't have them thinking it is the other person's job to protect them both. It is both their responsibilities. If they have information, they will be more prepared. They will also be free to say, "no" or "not at this time."

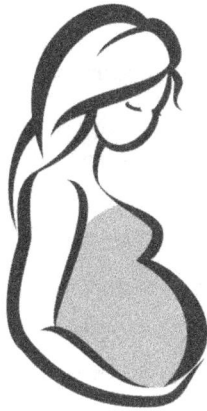

THINGS YOU CAN DO FOR
YOUR TEEN'S SUCCESS

Parents, do you wonder what your teen is thinking? Do you suddenly fell like you are living with a stranger? Does your teen tell you that you just don't understand? Here are some suggestions to help you help your teen.

First and foremost, remember YOU are the parent. The rules your teen lives by are yours. Set curfews and mean it. Set limits on phone time, computer time, video game time, and stick to them.

Secondly, make sure school work comes first. Be sure your teen is in school. Be sure there is a place to do homework. If your teen is having trouble with school work, find someone to help. The National Honor Society in your teen's high school might offer free tutoring.

Next, know when your teen is truly ready to date. Putting a thirteen-year-old in the car with teens who are sixteen and older might not be the wisest choice. Younger teens trying to fit in will be more likely to try different things to belong. Is a beer bad if you are not driving? The answer is, YES. How about other drugs? YES!!! Then of course, there is sex…NOT at thirteen.

If you are letting your teen date, set down rules. Make sure if there is a problem, your teen knows they can call you and you will come. Make sure your teen has a cell phone to use for the evening.

Teach your child etiquette for computer and cell phone use. Computers have become a good way for some teens to bully others. Teach your child the things which should and shouldn't be said in an instant message, text, or e-mail. Tell them the cell is only for emergencies. You do not expect them to be calling their friends. It should not be on in movie theaters or restaurants. If for some reason your child is going to miss curfew, it should be on. Text messaging is the same as computer use.

When using the Internet, be sure you know the sites your child is visiting. Chat rooms are not the best place for your teens. Use the parental block for sites you don't want them visiting. Some of the hottest sites are the most dangerous for teens. You need to be the Internet police in your home. Monitor the sites they go to and the game rooms they are in. Have their passwords so you can check up on them.

Routines are a must for teens. There should be a regular bed time. Take the TV out of the bedroom. Encourage TV watching with the family. Things for school should be put in the same place every night, so no one is racing around in the morning trying to find things. Mornings should start with a good breakfast. Time needs to be built in for breakfast. You don't have to cook a huge meal every day. There should be a set time for doing homework. It can be right after school or right after dinner, the choice is yours.

Talking with your teen needs to be a two-way conversation, not just you talking. You need to listen to what your teen is saying. Even if you don't like what you're hearing. Your teen needs to be able to voice their fears, concerns, opinions, and ask questions. You need to be calm when responding. Always stress honesty with your teen.

Take some time to be at the school. Check in with teachers and staff. Teen years are the ones where they need you the most and don't know how to ask.

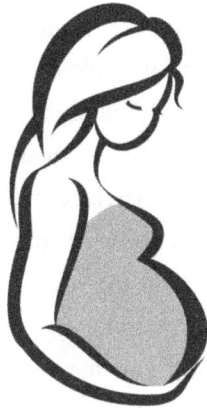

RESOURCES AND CLOSING NOTES

Here are some hotlines and websites:

- Birthright International
  1-800-550-4900 24hrs a day
  Birthright.org

- America's Crisis Pregnancy Helpline
  1-866-492-6466
  Thehelpline.org

- Bethany Christian Services
  1-800-238-4269
  Bethany.org

- CareNet
  1-703-554-8734
  care-net.org

- Option Line
  1-800-712-4357
  Optionline.org

These are a few places you can contact if you are uncomfortable speaking face-to-face or in your local community. This is by no means an inclusive list of all the places you could call. If you are in doubt, Google crisis pregnancy for access to phone numbers and agencies.

Are you prepared to become a statistic? Most women who have one baby without benefit of marriage live in poverty. Most of their children do, too. It is hard to break out of poverty once you are there. Is this the life you want for your child? Is this a risk you are willing to take?

Another statistic says if you have one child without marriage, you will most likely have one or two more. The cycle is vicious and continue to repeat itself. Think carefully before you put a baby into this situation.

Babies are NOT an answer to your problems. Find someone to talk to. Figure out what the problems are. Find solutions to the problems. Don't complicate things with a baby. Don't take the chance you will ruin lives, including yours. Get help and get it now.

You need to think everything through. Find someone to talk to whom you trust. Share your feelings with them. This is NOT a game. A baby is NOT a status symbol. It is NOT just your life, but also the lives of others. You CANNOT make a baby alone, so don't think you can raise one that way. Not all stories have happy endings.

A Public Service Reminder

Babies are for life. You don't get to turn them out at eighteen and tell them go forth and conquer the world. They will need to know they can always come home. Even when your babies marry and have children of their own, they are still your babies.

ABOUT THE AUTHOR

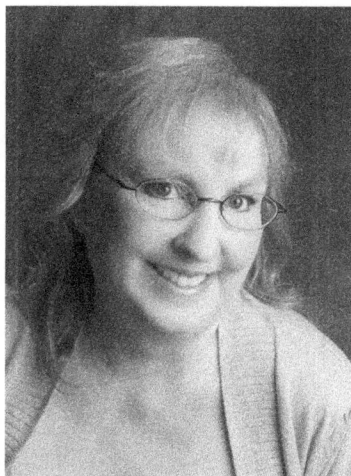

Retired teacher Rebecka Vigus spends her time writing, reading, crocheting, hiking, and swimming. She travels seeking the ideal place to call home. Ms. Vigus has been writing since she was in her pre-teens. Her first book was poetry, *Only a Start and Beyond*. Since then she has penned seven full-length novels, one book for children, and numerous short stories. Ms. Vigus has been listed as a Michigan Author and Illustrator at the State of Michigan website.

CPSIA information can be obtained
at www.ICGtesting.com
Printed in the USA
LVHW090916250420
654406LV00002B/626